TEMPTATION

TEMPTATION

BY JOHN WILLIAM GOOD

To order additional copies of this book, contact:
Xlibris Corporation
1-888-795-4274
www.Xlibris.com
Orders@Xlibris.com
116268

In the fall of 2006, after more than sixty years of good health, the temptation presented to Mary at a bus stop one morning finally caught up with her.

A visit to her gynecologist for her annual Pap smear showed an irregularity.

She was instructed to see a urologist immediately.

UROLOGY

10/16/06   Mary's urologist discovered a large tumor in Mary's bladder on or about October 16, 2006. A biopsy didn't show any sign of cancer cells.

The doctor scheduled a procedure to be performed on Monday, October 23, to have a better look at what he labeled as very suspicious. Mary's primary doctor was contacted to admit her for the procedure.

INTERNAL MEDICINE

10/18/06   On Wednesday, October 18, Mary's primary doctor discovered a problem with the carotid artery and scheduled an ultrasound.

10/19/06   The ultrasound was performed, and the scheduled procedure for Monday, the twenty-third, was cancelled with a CAT scan scheduled for Friday, the twentieth.

INTERVENTIONAL CARDIOLOGY, INTERNAL MEDICINE

10/25/06   MRI on Wednesday, the twenty-fifth, and a follow-up later in the day with the cardiologist. This doctor told Mary, one more cigarette and she could have a stroke or heart attack. She has not had one since.

Her *carotid artery* had a large amount of plaque buildup (90 percent blockage).

VASCULAR SURGERY, GENERAL SURGERY

10/26/06   An appointment with the carotid artery surgeon was set for October 26. He scheduled surgery for 11:00 AM, Monday, the thirtieth.

He also told us that Mary has a four-centimeter *abdominal aortic aneurysm* that we have to watch. If it reaches *five centimeters*, it will need attention. If she watches her *diet*, stays off *cigarettes*, and keeps the cholesterol under control, as well as her blood pressure, she could live her entire life without reaching the five centimeters. She is taking medications for blood pressure and cholesterol as well as one baby aspirin a day.

Table of Contents

Abdominal Aortic Aneurysm

Most abdominal aortic aneurysms (AAAs) are asymptomatic, not detectable on physical examination, and silent until discovered during radiologic testing for other reasons. Tobacco use, hypertension, a family history of AAA, and male sex are clinical risk factors for the development of an aneurysm. Ultrasound, the preferred method of screening, is cost-effective in high-risk patients. Repair is indicated when the aneurysm becomes greater than 5.5 cm in diameter or grows more than 0.6 to 0.8 cm per year. Asymptomatic patients with an AAA should be medically optimized before repair, including institution of beta blockade. Symptomatic aneurysms present with back, abdominal, buttock, groin, testicular, or leg pain and require urgent surgical attention. Rupture of an AAA involves complete loss of aortic wall integrity and is a surgical emergency requiring immediate repair. The mortality rate approaches 90 percent if rupture occurs outside the hospital. Although open surgical repair has been performed safely, an endovascular approach is used in select patients if the aortic and iliac anatomy are amenable. Two large randomized controlled trials did not find any improvement in mortality rate or morbidity with this approach compared with conventional open surgical repair. There is increased chance of rupture.

10/30/06   The surgery on the thirtieth was a success, and Mary is now ready for prep once again for the bladder procedure.

Description of Service:
RECHANNELING OF ARTERY
Date(s) of Service: 10/30/2006

11/06/06   Back to primary care doctor on the sixth of November

11/07/06   Then the cardiologist on the seventh of November

11/10/06   Mary's urologist performed the bladder procedure on Friday, the
            tenth. These pictures were from the urologist and are the actual
            tumor before and after.

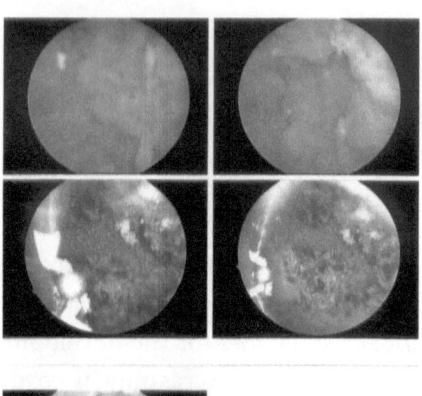

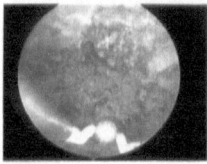

11/15/06   We met with the urologist on Wednesday, November 15, 2006,
            and he informed us it is cancer. But this type of cancer is rarely
            found in the bladder (lymphoepithelioma-like carcinoma), only
            eighty reported cases in the world. It is usually found in other
            parts of the body. The doctor said this is good news because
            there is a high success rate with this type of cancer.

Lymphoepithelioma-like carcinoma of the bladder consists of high-
grade tumor cells with syncytial appearance arranged in sheets and
anatomizing nests. In addition, there is strong suggestive evidence that
it responds to chemotherapy and there is the potential of salvaging the
bladder.

lymphoepithelioma (LIM-fo-EP-ih-THEE-lee-O-ma)
A type of cancer that begins in the tissues covering the nasopharynx (the
upper part of the throat behind the nose).

11/17/06   Friday, November 17, we met the oncologist, who said that is *good news* (I believe he said there is an 80 percent success rate with this type of cancer using chemotherapy) although they will have to call all over the world for help again because the cancer is in the bladder.

HEMATOLOGY/ONCOLOGY, INTERNAL MEDICINE

11/20/06   Mary had bone density testing on Monday the twentieth of November.

11/27/06   Mary has a PET scan on Monday, the twenty-seventh of November, to see if there is spreading (there has not been any indication of it spreading to other areas).

11-28-06   Met with the urologist on Tuesday, the twenty-eighth, to determine treatment and the extent of the treatment. Treatment will begin on Monday, December 4, 2006. There will be four treatments. Each treatment will be a week in duration. There will be two weeks between treatments resulting in telve weeks elapsed time. On the first day, chemo will be administered in the office for three hours (probably cisplatin). Then she will be outfitted with a pump, which will administer until Friday (probably fluorouracil), so two weeks between treatments.

Cisplatin is an anti-cancer ("antineoplastic" or "cytotoxic") chemotherapy drug. Cisplatin is classified as an "alkylating agent."

Used to treat testicular, ovarian, bladder, head and neck, esophageal, small and non-small cell lung, breast, cervical, stomach and prostate cancers. Also to treat Hodgkin's and non-Hodgkin's lymphomas, neuroblastoma, sarcomas, multiple myeloma, melanoma, and mesothelioma (http://www.chemocare.com/bio/cisplatin.asp).

Fluorouracil is an anti-cancer ("antineoplastic" or "cytotoxic") chemotherapy drug. Fluorouracil is classified as an "antimetabolite"

Colon and rectal cancer, Breast cancer, Gastrointestinal cancers including: anal, esphageal, pancreas and gastric (stomach), Head and neck cancer, Hepatoma (liver cancer), Ovarian cancer (http://www.chemocare.com/bio/fluorouracil.as).

Topical use (cream or solution) in basal cell cancer of the skin and actinic keratoses.

11-29-06   Appointment at one thirty with the urologist.

12-01-06 7:30 AM—blood work at Boca Raton Hospital.

TREATMENT

12-4-2006   A port was put in Mary's arm at 7:30 AM at the Boca Community Hospital. This port will remain until the treatments are finally over. It is used to replace the need of shots, etc. Everything will be input through the port, including the fluorouracil chemo drug.

On the first day, chemo (cisplatin) was administered at the oncology clinic for three hours. Then she was outfitted with a pump that will administer fluorouracil until Friday. The pump is connected to the port in her arm to allow the fluorouracil to flow into her bloodstream.

Mary was instructed to drink a lot of water and other liquids because the chemo drugs will dehydrate her badly. They said at least four twelve ounce bottles of water a day. At this point we do not know what to expect although we have heard horror stories about the treatment. She was told to expect to lose her hair. We had anticipated that and ordered a hairpiece back in November.

Date(s) of Service: 12/04/2006
automated hemogram
drawing blood

cisplatin, fifty-milligram injection (an anticancer drug)
fluorouracil injection (an anticancer drug)
dexamethasone sodium phosphate (a synthetic steroid and anti-
inflammatory drug)
interval history and examination
injection of heparin sodium per ten units <u>(anticoagulant)</u>
normal saline solution infusion

Date(s) of Service: 12/05/2006
fluorouracil injection (an anticancer drug)
interval history and examination
injection of heparin sodium per ten units (anticoagulant)
normal saline solution infusion
ondansetron HCl injection

Date(s) of Service: 12/07/2006
fluorouracil injection (an anticancer drug)
interval history and examination
injection of heparin sodium per ten units <u>(anticoagulant)</u>
normal saline solution infusion

1-1-2006 Pump was removed and Mary was hydrated because she was not
drinking enough water. She also has not eaten since the chemo
began on Monday, December 4, and she is getting very weak.

Date(s) of Service: 12/08/2006
injection of heparin sodium per ten units (anticoagulant)

Mary's daughter, Stephanie, came on Friday, the eighth, for the
weekend. We bought sandwiches at Jersey Sub, a chicken salad
for Mary, but she hardly touched it.

1-1-2006 We went with Mary's daughter, Stephanie, to the flea market on
Sample Road. Mary was weak but managed to make it, being the
trooper she is.

1-1-2006 We had an early Christmas dinner at home, turkey and all the
fixings. Mary touched her turkey but ate very little.

1-1-2006   Back to oncology clinic for more hydration. Stephanie went shopping; we picked up some Dunkin' Donuts, but Mary only took a bite of her favorite bow tie. Stephanie left at 4:00 PM to go back to New Hampshire. Mary was now weak and could not even go to the airport with her.

Date(s) of Service: 12/11/2006
automated hemogram
drawing blood

1-1-2006   We had called the oncology clinic to report the drinking and eating problems. We needed the Lakehouse wheelchair due to her weakness of legs. The urologist was not very happy, said he is giving her a very heavy dose to try to save the bladder; we should have told him earlier. They hydrated her again.

Date(s) of Service: 12/13/2006
automated hemogram
drawing blood
interval history and examination
injection of heparin sodium per ten units (anticoagulant)
normal saline solution infusion

12-14-2006 She ate a little Jell-O and tapioca pudding today.

12-15-2006 Back to the oncology clinic, more hydration, blood work, etc.

Date(s) of Service: 12/15/2006
interval history and examination
injection of heparin sodium per ten units (anticoagulant)
normal saline solution infusion

12-17-2006 It is Sunday morning, and I awoke to Mary having her Christmas turkey.

12-18-2006 Mary went to work today.

12-20-2006 Back to oncology clinic for more blood work. She went with her friend Mary Stout to the Outback and ate a complete steak dinner. She also worked four days this week.

Date(s) of Service: 12/20/2006
automated hemogram
drawing blood

1-1-2006   TenetCare, part of West Boca Medical Center for blood work in preparation for a blood transfusion tomorrow. Chemo has killed red blood cells.

1-1-2006   About six hours at the West Boca Medical Center for blood transfusion.

1-1-2006   Hair missing, we picked up hairpiece. Can't tell the difference.

12-24-2006 We went to the 10:30 PM services at Bethesda by the Sea in West Palm. Got home about twelve thirty. She held up well but was real tired.

12-26-06   Second chemo treatment scheduled to start. However, swelling started in Mary's feet and ankles. Clinic decided to postpone the *cisplatin* until cause could be determined. The pump is connected to the port in her arm to allow the *fluorouracil* to flow into her bloodstream.

Date(s) of Service: 12/26/2006
automated hemogram
drawing blood
fluorouracil injection
dexamethasone sodium phosphate (a synthetic steroid and anti-inflammatory drug)
injection of heparin sodium per ten units (anticoagulant)
normal saline solution infusion

12-27-2006 Mary actually went to work today, wearing the pump and new hair (her boss thought it was her hair). Appetite and liquid intake are normal. She was told by phone that the swelling was caused by the blood transfusion.

12-28-2006 Back to oncology clinic and administration of the cisplatin. We picked up a steak on the way home so she could get a headstart on the appetite loss coming. She ate about half of her steak and a few Boston baked beans before the drug stole her appetite.

Date(s) of Service: 12/28/2006
cisplatin, fifty-milligram injection
interval history and examination
fluorouracil injection
dexamethasone sodium phosphate (a synthetic steroid and anti-inflammatory drug)
injection of heparin sodium per ten units (anticoagulant)
normal saline solution infusion
furosemide injection (a drug used to treat excessive fluid accumulation)

12-29-2006 Pump removed at oncology clinic and some other tests performed. They told Mary there would be six treatments instead of four. Obviously disheartening news, but she is handling it.

From the oncology clinic to see the urologist at ten thirty. He wanted to look inside for a status but instead rescheduled the look-see for January 10.

Appetite is gone, only eating about one-half serving of chicken and noodle soup a day (eight ounces, maybe). Water doesn't work anymore, makes her sick, drinks mostly ginger ale. Still trying Jell-O once in a while.

12-30-2006 Cisplatin has taken over. She had a little soup and lost it; water not good either. We will look for another liquid.

1-1-2007 To oncology clinic for shot for hemoglobin and white blood cells. Very weak, wanted wheelchair because of legs. Not available, so she was able to walk successfully.

automated hemogram
drawing blood

We are searching for the right liquid now. Ginger ale still works. To the store and bought cranberry juice cocktail, cran-grape, and cran-apple. They seem to work. We are having an awful time finding Popsicles though.

1-1-2007   Mary is still not eating. Yesterday we tried bologna—no good. Today I went and bought baby food; maybe she had a little applesauce. She is able to eat the chicken noodle soup, but tonight she told me she now cannot eat the chicken chunks in the soup.

Decision is made that if she doesn't start eating tomorrow, we call the doctor, probably will admit her into hospital, where they can get some food in. She is losing weight too fast. Sleeps a lot, no energy, and of course, in the past few days, has the leg problems. Weight is now at 110, much too low.

1-1-2007   Mary had about half an egg, a couple of pieces of potato, and a little toast. Then at 4:00 PM we went to the Outback, where she ate about three ounces of steak, a little of her baked potato, one piece of brown bread, and a little of her salad.

1-1-2007   Mary finished off the Outback dinner this morning (about six ounces of steak and a baked potato) then went for about a two-hour nap. Her legs still bother her unless she takes pain pills. She wanted to go to work but was still not up to it.

1-1-2007   At 11:00 AM, we went to the oncology clinic. Mary ate soup, a slice of pizza, and half a sub sandwich.

automated hemogram
drawing blood

1-1-2007   Appointment at nine thirty with Mary's urologist, had CAM look at bladder and three biopsies.

The urology office called to say the urine was clear.

1-1-2007   Mary's urologist called (on a Saturday), excited to tell Mary that the biopsies came back negative, cancer hasn't penetrated.

1-1-2007   Mary went to work back on a full-day schedule but couldn't make the whole day.

1-1-2007   Oncology appointment then to work. Left work at around three thirty (taxi).

1-1-2007   Port in Mary's arm is infected. She was sent to the hospital to have it looked at. At the Boca Community Hospital, fluid was removed from infection and sent to be cultured. Results in about two days; Mary is to take more antibiotics until results are known. May have to remove port. Chemo is probably on hold until this is cleared up. Called her boss and told him he will have to get someone else, she cannot work.

Physician:
puncture drainage of lesion
echo guide for biopsy

01-23-2007   Chemo treatment 3 started today after infection cleared

automated hemogram
drawing blood
cisplatin, fifty-milligram injection (an anticancer drug)
fluorouracil injection (an anticancer drug)
dexamethasone sodium phosphate (a synthetic steroid and anti-inflammatory drug)
interval history and examination
injection of heparin sodium per ten units (anticoagulant)
normal saline solution infusion

01-25-2007   fluorouracil injection (an anticancer drug)
interval history and examination
injection of heparin sodium per ten units (anticoagulant)
normal saline solution infusion

01-26-2007   interval history and examination
             injection of heparin sodium per ten units (anticoagulant)
             normal saline solution infusion

01-29-2007   White blood cell shot today.

             filgrastim 480-microgram injection

01-30-2007   Needed the wheelchair to get to and from the lobby today. Ten
             o'clock appointment at the oncology clinic. The oncologist wants
             to see Mary on the fifth, concerned with her body's reaction.
             May delay the next two chemos.

             automated hemogram
             drawing blood

             Made American chop suey today, and she ate about eight ounces.
             Also picked up McDonald's shake, and she drank half.

02-12-2007   Chemo treatment number 4 started; this may be the last.

             automated hemogram
             drawing blood
             cisplatin, fifty-milligram injection (an anticancer drug)
             fluorouracil injection (an anticancer drug)
             dexamethasone sodium phosphate (a synthetic steroid and anti-
             inflammatory drug)
             interval history and examination
             injection of heparin sodium per ten units (anticoagulant)
             normal saline solution infusion

02-14-2007   fluorouracil injection (an anticancer drug)

02-16-2007   Needed wheelchair both ways. As she was very dehydrated, the
             clinic hydrated her.

             interval history and examination
             injection of heparin sodium per ten units (anticoagulant)
             normal saline solution infusion

02-18-2007 Mary had the worst weekend yet, real sick, hardly able to move around, stayed in bed most of the time.

02-19-2007 Reaction is worst it has been to date. Wheelchairs needed on both ends, blood pressure real low (causing dizziness)—she was told to stop blood pressure medicine. Hydrated twice. The oncologist is very concerned with her local health, will cut back dose or maybe stop altogether. Mary had a little chicken noodle soup in the evening, and a little Jell-O later. Drinking cranberry-grape juice.

automated hemogram
drawing blood
dexamethasone sodium phosphate (a synthetic steroid and anti-inflammatory drug)
interval history and examination
injection of heparin sodium per ten units (anticoagulant)
normal saline solution infusion
dolasetron mesylate (prevents nausea and vomiting that may be caused by cancer, blocks the serotonin pathway by which chemotherapy stimulates the vomiting center in the brain)

02-20-2007 Call from the oncology clinic. They need to do more lab work on Wednesday, check kidney functions, etc. Made an appointment for 8:45 AM. Mary had some Boost today to try and get some nutrients, lost it about an hour later. Drinking cranberry-apple juice.

02-21-2007 Still needs the wheelchair in both directions. More hydration in addition to lab work.

automated hemogram
drawing blood
interval history and automated hemogram
drawing blood
dexamethasone sodium phosphate (a synthetic steroid and anti-inflammatory drug)
interval history and examination

injection of heparin sodium per ten units (anticoagulant)
normal saline solution infusion
dolasetron mesylate (prevents nausea and vomiting that may
be caused by cancer, blocks the serotonin pathway by which
chemotherapy stimulates the vomiting center in the brain)
normal saline solution infusion
ondansetron HCl injection (serotonin 5-HT receptor antagonist
used mainly to treat nausea and vomiting following chemotherapy).

02-22-2007   Using wheelchair both ways still. More hydration today. Also, potassium level down, prescription filled to improve. Need to return tomorrow.

interval history and examination
normal saline solution infusion
injection of heparin sodium per ten units (anticoagulant)

02-23-2007   To oncology again today and again wheelchair needed in both directions. She is, however, a little stronger. This time, the mouth and throat are the biggest problems and, of course, not able to eat. Appointment again on Monday, the twenty-sixth. This is the eleventh day, and so far she usually doesn't start eating until the twelfth or thirteenth day.

automated hemogram
drawing blood
dexamethasone sodium phosphate (a synthetic steroid and anti-inflammatory drug)
injection of heparin sodium per ten units (anticoagulant)
normal saline solution infusion
dolasetron mesylate (**prevents nausea and vomiting that may be caused by cancer, blocks the serotonin pathway by which chemotherapy stimulates the vomiting center in the brain**)

1-1-2007   To oncology and again the wheelchair needed in both directions. Met with the oncologist, and he said she will be 100 percent and there will be no more chemotherapy. If she doesn't improve by tomorrow, she will need to be hospitalized. He wants her to drink four bottles of Boost a day and suggests mixing a little ice cream in with it. We bought ice cream on the way home, and she drank a bottle of Boost at 1:00 PM. When I came home from work at 10:30 PM, she informed me she had lost the Boost at 5:00 PM.

automated hemogram
drawing blood
interval history and examination
injection of heparin sodium per ten units (anticoagulant)
normal saline solution infusion

1-1-2007   Mary called the oncologist and said she was ready to go to the hospital. Admitted her to Boca Community at around 11:30 AM. She will probably be there for a couple of days.

1-1-2007   Visited Mary at Boca Community, room 819, at 11:00 AM. She improved just a little. She said they had kept her up all night with tests, etc. She had a chest x-ray and a blood transfusion. Told me she had part of a muffin for breakfast, but the mouth and throat still very sore. Mary's oncologist had been in to see her. Blood pressure was taken while I visited, and it was back to normal.

1-1-2007   Visit with Mary at the hospital around 11:00 AM. She is improved today, a little stronger, had a regular lunch delivered while I was there (she complained about lack of salt, pepper, and butter). I brought her the orange soda (flat) she requested, some chocolate boost and some books to read. She says they may release her on the weekend. Mary's primary care doctor had been in to see her. He said she should stay off the blood pressure medicine for a little while. Sign on the door is telling me to check with nurse station before entering. This was because of chance for infection or a virus, cold, etc.

1-1-2007   Scheduled to leave the hospital at noon, but due to some lab foul-ups, we didn't get out until after 3:00 PM. Mary is still very weak but is happy to be home. We stopped at the Boca Diner for her favorite turkey dinner, but when we got home, she couldn't eat it. We needed the wheelchair at home.

1-1-2007   We made a trip to Publix to check blood pressure (106 over 77), and Mary called it in to the oncologist. Mary ate a little chicken noodle soup and a small muffin. Later while I was at work, she drank a Boost. She needed the wheelchair going and coming.

1-1-2007   I awoke early, determined Mary was going to eat. I cooked bacon and eggs with an English muffin and some orange juice. She ate half of the muffin, drank the orange juice, and ate one slice of bacon and the egg. We then went to the oncology clinic, where the oncologist said he is pleased with her progress. She weighs 107 pounds today. A PET scan is scheduled for 8:00 AM on March 22 at the imaging center of the Boca Raton Community Hospital. This should tell us if it is all gone or not.

After the clinic, Mary drank a bottle of Boost. Then before I left for work, she had a peach quarter and a little Jell-O. I prepared her turkey dinner, but she wasn't up to that yet. She tires easily but did get around today without the use of a wheelchair.

1-1-2007   Another small gain in energy and wellness noticed today, and Mary said she felt just slightly better. She had about one fourth of the turkey dinner and a chocolate Boost before I left for work.

1-1-2007   Breakfast around 9:30 AM. She ate well, an egg, a waffle, and one slice of bacon. However, she lost it about half an hour later. Nausea is still a problem.

NOTE: Many people with good intentions keep calling. One lady called three times yesterday. They just don't seem to understand why Mary doesn't want to talk. Everyone in the family and all her friends seem to get the picture and honor my request to call me first. When I am home, I keep her phone, but when I have to leave for work, she needs the phone in case she needs to call me. I am not the one with this dreadful disease; I am just an onlooker, but I can see with my own eyes why she doesn't want to talk to anyone. She is a very sick girl with just one wish, for all the sickness to go away.

1-1-2007   Mary is very depressed today because of losing her breakfast yesterday. I suspect I fed her too much on her first day back to some real food. Today I fed in little bits and pieces, a couple of small meatballs, then later, a little spaghetti (maybe a tablespoon plus) with a couple of meatballs and a little sauce. Tried to get Ensure into her, but she wasn't having any today.

1-1-2007   I nagged her today to eat. I bought some fruits in juices, but nothing appealed. I suspect the lack of appetite is encouraged by the depression over the nausea. I did manage to influence a couple of bottles of Ensure (350 calories each), and she tried a little of the fruit. I also had bought fresh strawberries, and she had one with sugar on it.

1-1-2007   Appointment at the oncology clinic with the oncologist at nine forty-five. We needed the wheelchair, and when he saw her in the chair, he was quite bothered. He said she must eat, she must call him tomorrow at 9:00 AM, and that if she isn't better, he will have to put her in the hospital again, which he does not want to do. They gave some intravenous fluids, which gave her energy, and she left without the wheelchair. Also did not use the wheelchair back at Lakehouse. Once in the apartment, she had two cups of Campbell's special chicken and noodle soup and finished off the can of Ensure she started before going to the clinic. Calorie intake so far today then is about 180 for the soup and 350 for the Ensure as of 2:00 PM. Her weight was 105 today, another 2-pound loss.

1-1-2007   We tried oatmeal this morning—she couldn't keep it down, probably the milk. She resolved to drink only Ensure, depressed even more. Mary called me at work around 7:00 PM, depressed, said she couldn't do what her oncologist had asked, drink four Ensures a day. I told her she has to, and when I got home, she had drunk about three.

1-1-2007   I persuaded her to have a little tomato soup around 10:00 AM, and she drank a can of ginger ale. At eleven thirty I made a grilled cheese and she ate almost one fourth of the sandwich and a little (very little) more tomato soup. Just before I left for work at one forty-five, she had another Ensure.

03-16-2007 Today Mary was off eating again. She had a little American chop suey and more Ensure.

03-17-2007 She ate most of an egg, half an English muffin, and a small piece of London broil steak, with a little of my special five-second breakfast drink, which consists of banana, orange juice, and yogurt. An Ensure later and one fourth of a grilled cheese.

03-18-2007 Today started with a small piece of top of round steak and one egg. This was followed about two hours later with a bottle of Ensure. At around 4:00 PM, we tried some red bean soup, but no luck there. Mary is convinced she will never get her taste buds back to normal. However, she will be going on an errand with me tomorrow to West Palm Beach. Progress is slow. It has been thirty days now since the last chemotherapy treatment stopped. Her hemoglobin and platelets are normal, so she is recovering, just this problem with eating.

03-19-2007 This morning, Mary went with me on an errand to West Palm Beach, Virginia. It was her longest outing during this period other than doctor's visits. We stopped to buy some fresh melon pieces on the way back. She drank a bottle of Ensure during the trip. However, when we got home, the fresh fruit did not stay with her. She had another Ensure. I left her with a fresh bottle of water and more Ensure when I went to work at 2:00 PM. We needed the wheelchair in both directions since she is still very weak.

03-20-2007 Nohing much new today. Mary basically decided to stick with the Ensure and had already three bottles by 2:00 PM. The only solid she tried was a little fruit at lunchtime. Her reasoning was fear of vomiting.

03-21-2007 More improvement today. By noon Mary had eaten one half of a grilled cheese and tomato sandwich, had a little red bean soup, one Ensure, and one Boost. Also drinking some water and sodas. She says taste is still not the same, but a little taste has returned. This is the most improvement I have seen for a while. Tomorrow is a big day, PET scan, but I don't know when we will get the results.

03-22-2007 Every day is just a little better. We needed the wheelchair for leaving and returning to Lakehouse, but she walked at the hospital for her PET scan. The scan was supposed to take two hours, instead took two and a half hours (left her a little tired). On the way home she suggested Kentucky Fried Chicken, which we bought. She ate about half a breast, quite a bit of meat, and one serving of potatoes with gravy and maybe a tablespoon of peas. Unfortunately, she lost some of it but wasn't discouraged this time because it was just a little and she had a little taste of the chicken. Gives her hope that her buds will be back. She said when this is over, she is hitting every restaurant on Federal Highway.

03-23-2007 A bigger step toward recovery today, I think. We bought a whole chicken at the fresh market, and she ate a considerable portion with a baked potato and peas. When I left at 2:00 PM, she had not become sick. She also had some fresh melon, which stayed with her. We are waiting with bated breath for the results of yesterday's PET scan.

03-24-2007 Even bigger steps today, had a good breakfast, egg, bacon, french toast, and orange juice. Later, chicken, baked potato, and peas. Then a desert of upside-down cake. A little upset stomach around 10:00 PM, but nothing serious. A lot more energy today, hope she didn't over do it.

03-25-2007 This cancer treatment recovery is a tough go. Today was not as good as yesterday; she is listless with very little appetite. Yesterday she was full of energy early in the day—today, not so all day. She did have some macaroni and cheese, a few sodas, and a little harvest cake. Hopefully, tomorrow will be a better day.

Weight is down to one hundred today.

03-26-2007 Back to improvements today. I awoke to Mary fixing breakfast, bacon and french toast with orange juice. Later around noon, she had Stouffers macaroni and cheese. I spoke with her at 5:00 PM from work, and she was beginning to fade. She called the oncologist for any news on the PET scan but as of 5:00 PM had not heard from him.

03-27-2007 Another day of gain. Mary was up early and cleaning and cooking. Energy I take as a good sign. She made a baked macaroni and cheese she saw on TV, and she ate some Stouffers. Also one complete hamburger with a few baked beans. Her taste hasn't returned yet, but at least she is eating.

03-28-2007 Mary didn't have the energy or appetite she has had the last couple of days. When I questioned, she only said she needs her taste buds back to eat. But she did have some chicken, a baked potato, and peas.

Mary's oncologist called around noon to tell her the results of the PET scan were great and now she must see the urologist for a CAM look inside again. It looks real promising for her.

03-29-2007 Today, as yesterday, we started the day with a Dunkin' Donut bow tie. Yesterday she ate the whole thing, but today without taste buds working, she only managed three-fourths of it. She did, however, have some Kraft macaroni and cheese for lunch. Later in the day, she had a cheeseburger for supper.

A doctor at work gave me some great input for two urologists if we need a second opinion or other services. One of them is the head of urology at Miami. She said they are hard to get an appointment with, but she has connections and will help us if the need arises. The other urologist was from Fort Lauderdale. One of the things this illness has done is show the kindness of people all around us.

We have an appointment with Mary's oncologist, Monday morning, April 2. We should have a pretty good feel for what to expect next after that visit. Right now the big thing seems to be the absence of taste, and we can only hope it returns soon.

03-30-2007 Mary slept late this morning but got up hungry. She had an egg, some bacon, and french toast. She tasted it a little, maybe because she cooked, instead of me. She has, however, had a rather blah day as of 6:00 PM, was listless, and couldn't seem to get interested in food. She said she tried some tomato soup, but no go.

Her legs are still pretty weak and her energy level is low, but all in all she is progressing, although slow.

03-31-2007 A little more energy today. Went with me to check out Chinese food and later to pick up a pizza. Note that Chinese food was horrible. Anyway, it looks like she is getting a little of her taste back.

04-03-2007 Appetite and energy level continue to improve. Yesterday, April 2, she had an appointment with the oncologist. He is pleased with her recovery, and she had gained six pounds of what she had lost. On the sixteenth she will be seen by her urologist to have a look at the bladder again.

Today she had an active day, prepared and sent Easter cards, went to the post office for stamps, and did a little of her own grocery shopping, admitting to me just before I left for work that she had actually run out of steam at the market but still she pushed on. Steak and beans for lunch, and she is getting some of her taste buds back.

04-08-2007 Easter Sunday 2007, and Mary was up early preparing for church. We drove up to Bethesda in Palm Beach for the 9:00 AM service. We were back home about eleven thirty, and she was still holding up well.

After a small breakfast, some Portuguese bread, juice, coffee, etc., she took a short nap. Then up and at it cooking an Easter dinner with a honey-baked ham and all the trimmings. But after dinner she was feeling low and off to bed to get back some of that energy. She is probably more frustrated now than depressed because she tires so easily. But her body has taken a real beating these past few months, and it will be a while before she fully recovers.

However, she looks great with good color and skin condition. I think when she is back, she will be better than ever.

Mary does take a phone call once in a while now, but please be patient with her; sometimes she is just not up to talking, and I told her, "Don't answer then." I am sure everyone understands.

04-13-2007 Mary still has not recovered her taste buds, and although everything we read says her hair should have started to grow back in two to three weeks, it has been two months and there has been no sign of that happening yet. Furthermore, I had to instruct her that she cannot use chemicals on her new hair. No wonder she is a little depressed these days. She is cooking up a storm, trying every food for some taste. We tried several Chinese and seafood places but only found a close taste for fish and chips at an English pub. She ate everything but said only because it looked like it tasted good. She did, however, taste a sip of my beer.

Monday, the sixteenth, is a big day when another internal exam will check the status of cancer, gone or not? Then the next day she meets with the oncologist. She expects him to want more procedures but with radiation. He called his contacts in Italy, and that is what they are suggesting. She obviously doesn't want anything, but the two doctors will decide what is best.

Today she had a call from the doctor of vascular and endovascular surgery that performed the carotid artery surgery. I assume he wants an appointment to check that status as well as a look at the aneurysm. She has two appointments next week, so she said she will call him next week. She is understandably tired of sickness and doctors. One concern is that she hasn't been able to take her blood pressure and cholesterol medicine during the chemotherapy, and they are important to her other health.

04-18-2007 The checkup with the urologist went well on Monday. He did three biopsies and said everything looks good but he will call when the biopsy result comes back. If the biopsy is negative, he will then want another hospital visit for some more scraping just to make sure. In the meantime he scheduled the next appointment for three months and said that will continue for at least a year.

On the home front, on Saturday we drove up and down Federal Highway Delray to Boca Raton, tasting a slice of pizza at every shop we could find. Still trying to the taste buds back.

On Tuesday at the oncology clinic, everything looked good; she got a shot of something, and her weight was at 117.

04-20-2007 Mary's urologist called around 10:00 AM today to tell Mary the biopsies done Monday came back negative. He spoke with her oncologist, and they think she may have beaten the cancer. She will still need one more trip to the hospital for a thorough internal examination, but for now everything looks *great!*

04-21-2007 With great news yesterday, it just keeps getting better. Today she is tasting food better, and yes—hair is starting to grow back.

05-01-2007 Mary saw the urologist on April 16 when he took the biopsies that allowed him to call on Friday, following that he thinks she has beaten the cancer; of course, no one really knows for sure. He said he wanted to perform the same procedure that he performed on November 10 last year to make sure all is well.

On April 27, Mary saw her oncologist, and he encouraged her to have the procedure done. She had been hesitating and questioning the need. She, however, will have it done on May, the eighth.

Today she saw her primary care doctor after having a chest x-ray on April 30 as part of the pre-op for her hospital visit on May 8. He cleared her for the procedure.

Mary will see the surgeon who cleared her carotid artery on October 30, 2006, on May 15. He needs to check the artery as well as the aneurysm.

05-11-2007   Mary continues to receive good reports. On Tuesday, May 8, 2007, she had a procedure at the Boca Raton Community Hospital to look into the bladder for any remaining traces of the cancer, and the first report from a very happy urologist was she is clean. We are still waiting for the results of biopsies taken at that procedure.

She has gained enough weight to begin thinking about salads again.

05-22-2007   Mary had the port removed from her arm. Her comment was "Now the nightmare is over." She, of course, still must have regular checkups and watch herself, but for now she appears to be out of the woods.

06-02-2007   we have sold our home in Florida and are returning to New England. We will be leaving here, God willing, on June 11 and be in our new home on June 15, 2007. Mary seems to have recovered well from the cancer and other ailments she had, but we will seek a second opinion once back in Boston.

06-03-2007   Mary had some blood work today, which means a call to the Urologist tomorrow. That cancer is a scary thing.

06-04-2007   urologist says everything looks normal. He will talk to new doctor when we get to Boston.

06-14-2007   We moved from Boca Raton, Florida, to our new home in Hudson, New Hampshire.

07-05-2007 It became necessary to have some lab work done regarding the cancer, and we went to a hospital in Nashua, New Hampshire. The hospital refused to treat Mary. We called Mary's doctor in Florida, and he placed an order for lab work to be done at the Nashua hospital. That lab work was *never* returned to the doctor in Florida; in fact, the hospital sent it to some doctor in Massachusetts. The cancer has subsequently returned. Although we are sure the hospital would deny any fault in this matter and certainly we cannot be sure whether or not the refusal had anything to do with the return, it is equally certain that early detection is of benefit, and that just may have played a part. In any case, we only have one concern, Mary's health, which we have already put in the hands of Dana-Farber, where she will certainly not be refused.

07-31-2007 finally, after several weeks we now have Mary set up with medical care at Dana-Farber and Brigham and Women's in Boston. Yesterday, July 30, she met with an oncologist, and we were both impressed. He immediately began finding her a primary care doctor and a urologist. She will be seeing both real soon. They as a group will review all her records forwarded from Florida, which also was a difficult task to obtain. Amazing how the doctors in Florida just sort of said she's gone, good luck to her. It is difficult to get any cooperation from the offices in Florida. The doctors at Dana-Farber have frightened Mary with thoughts of radiation treatment but are not so sure the cancer is completely gone after such a small treatment.

08-02-2007 Mary now has a full complement of doctors.

Chief of the urology division at Brigham and Women's Hospital. Her first appointment is on Wednesday, August 8.

An appointment is set with a primary care doctor for August, the twenty-third.

Both are at Brigham and Women's Hospital, connected to Dana-

Farber. Really great to only have to go to one location for all medicals, and one of the best at that.

08-08-2007 Mary had her appointment with the urologist today. We were both impressed with his professionalism and manner. He went over the records sent from Florida and confirmed she had a very rare cancer. When Mary asked him if he had seen this type, he said only one such case, and therefore he had to do some research before we met today. He feels at this point that radiation and/or surgery is not needed. She should be checked every three months.

Mary has a CT scan scheduled for Friday, the seventeenth of August, just after she sees her new primary care doctor. The urologist will do a cystoscopy on August 21 to have a look at the bladder. I believe he said the CT scan should be done every six months.

08-21-2007 the cystoscopy was performed today, and the urologist said everything looks good. He said the CT scan showed the same results. He reiterated the need for an appointment in late November for another cystoscopy and one every three months thereafter. He also said a CT scan should be done again in six months but to check with the oncologist on that.

08-23-2007 Mary met with her new primary care doctor. She had a Pap smear and scheduled a colonoscopy for October 23 with a Dr. Poneros. Also scheduled a mammo on November 27, 2007. She said to speak with the oncologist about the CT scan and to see her in six months. The aorta aneurysm has grown to 4.6 centimeters and should be checked again in six months. The surgeon in Boca had said she is safe up to 5 centimeters.

08-24-2007 at 9:00 AM the oncologist called to inform Mary the CAT scan showed another mass, not on the bladder, and they will have to schedule a procedure to do a biopsy of the mass.

09-10-2007 the world is full of surprises, not all of them good. Today we got a bad one. The cancer has spread. Mary is scheduled for several scans on September 21 at Dana-Farber for the brain, the bone, and the chest. After that we will know more about the prognosis. For now she is obviously in shock. The oncologist said it does not look good but because the chemo worked well before, there is some hope it will work well again. I will be posting the blogs when we hear anything. What I need to concentrate on now is keeping her spirits up and helping her to fight this thing. And we need all the prayers we can get. { What is metastasis? Metastasis means the spread of cancer. Cancer cells can break away from a primary tumor and enter the bloodstream or lymphatic system (the tissues and organs that produce, store, and carry the cells that fight infections). That is how cancer cells spread to other parts of the body. Cancer cells may spread to lymph nodes (rounded masses of lymphatic tissue) near the primary tumor (regional lymph nodes). This is called lymph node involvement, positive nodes, or regional disease. Cancer that spreads to other organs or to lymph nodes far from the primary tumor is called metastatic disease or distant disease. When cancer cells spread and form a new tumor in a different organ, the new tumor is a metastatic tumor. The cancer cells in the metastatic tumor are like those in the original tumor. That means, for example, that if breast cancer spreads to the lung, the metastatic tumor in the lung is made up of abnormal breast cells (not abnormal lung cells). The disease in the lung is metastatic breast cancer (not lung cancer). Under a microscope, breast cancer cells look the same whether they are found in the breast or have spread to another part of the body. Metastatic cancers may be found before or at the same time as the primary tumor, or months or years later. When a new tumor is found in a patient who has been treated for cancer in the past, it is more often a metastasis than another primary tumor.}

09-12-2007 I spoke with the oncologist today. I had asked him for a further explanation of what "It doesn't look good" meant. As I suspected it simply meant the cancer had metastasized, not that all hope was lost. I asked him where it had spread, and he said it is in two lymph nodes near the bladder. He confirmed my suspicions that the further tests were to ascertain whether or not it had spread to other areas. He has already met with the urologist and has a backup plan if chemo doesn't work this time (but feels that since it worked before, there is a good chance it will work again). The backup plan is surgery. Of course, if it has spread to other areas, the plan will need revision. The oncologist also spoke with Mary and calmed her fears a little (in the above discussion of metastasis, you will see the use of lymph nodes in the spread of the cancer).

09-21-2007 the September 21 tests have been completed: brain scan, bone scan, CT scan, left-knee scan. Mary had bumped herself in the chest last week, and that bruise showed up in the scans. We won't know anything about the results until sometime next week.

09-26-2007 Mary had a consultation with the oncologist today to discuss the results of all the testing. He reiterated that nothing new had been found but for her to get ready for another roller coaster. He told her the chemotherapy will start next week, October 5, and again on October 11. If it doesn't work, there will be nothing more they can do for her. That is contrary to what he told us last week when he said he had met with Mary's urologist and they had a backup plan.

10-01-2007 I called the urologist for a further explanation and received the following e-mail, "The Urologist has reviewed the Oncologist note from Mrs. Good's visit with him on September 26th. It looks like surgery will not be an option at this time. The Urologist suggests that you be in touch with a new Oncologist at Dana-Farber. The new Oncologist should be able to address all of your questions regarding Mrs. Good's treatment."

10-05-2007 Mary's chemotherapy started today: five hours of infusion, three hours of cisplatin, and two hours of Gemzar. Four to six three-week cycles are expected. A cycle will be week 1, the cisplatin Gemzar, a five-hour infusion; second week will be one hour infusion of Gemzar; and the third week, nothing. We spoke with the nurse practitioner today and resolved some of the questions regarding the confusion about surgery as a backup. The chemo is supposed to shrink the size of the tumor, if not get rid of it completely. If it doesn't get rid of it or shrink it, then surgery would be out of the question and the plan changes to taking care of her as opposed to working for a cure. The general feeling is that since the chemo worked before, it will again. She did say that if they had felt it wouldn't work, there would not have even been chemo. Not the most encouraging words, but that's cancer! Cisplatin is an anticancer ("antineoplastic" or "cytotoxic") chemotherapy drug. Cisplatin is classified as an "alkylating agent." Gemzar is an anticancer ("antineoplastic" or "cytotoxic") chemotherapy drug. Gemzar is classified as an antimetabolite. Gemzar is given by infusion through a vein (intravenously, by IV). There is no pill form of Gemzar. The amount of Gemzar you will receive depends on many factors, including your height and weight, your general health or other health problems, and the type of cancer you have.

10-25-2007 we both liked Mary's new oncologist very much. He explained everything in good detail. The chemo cycle for today had to be postponed because her white blood cell count was bad, as was the hemoglobin. The cycle will start next week, then after the second week she will need a shot to make sure the white blood cell count and hemoglobin problem doesn't occur again. She had the same problem last year and had to have a blood transfusion. They are really alert here. This doctor explained the possible consequences if the chemo does not work and also explained there are no promises. He said nothing Mary did caused the cancer; she was just unlucky. If the chemo does not work, they will change directions, and they have a pill to maintain enabling living with cancer. Mary told him that yesterday she had a small pain in the area of the cancer. He said that could mean the chemo was working and the tumor was getting smaller, or it could mean it wasn't and the tumor was growing. In any case, at the end of this next cycle, she will have a CAT scan do see just what is happening. The next cycle will start then on November 1 with the second a week later, on the eighth. At this point the CAT scan is scheduled on the sixteenth of November, and she will probably see the doctor on Thanksgiving week and more than likely start the third cycle that day or at least have some kind of answers.

11-01-2007   the second of six cycles began today without incident. Mary's white cell count was back to normal. However, she had some kind of vision loss after arriving, thus causing a CT scan to try to find out the cause. Chances are it was just nerves. She will have the second phase of this second cycle on the eighth then a booster shot on the ninth to protect the white count during this cycle. Then on November 16, she will have a CT scan to determine if the chemotherapy is doing its job, shrinking the tumor.

11-08-2007   the second phase of the second cycle of chemotherapy began today with an early morning trip to Boston in twenty-four-degree weather. We really did not freeze. Mary had her IV fitted at 8:00 AM followed with a meeting with the nurse practitioner. We found out the CT scan she had last week due to the fog she encountered showed everything normal (that was a brain scan, not the one expected to check her progress). We discussed the progress scan, and it looks like it may be done after the third cycle, which will begin on the twenty-third, the day after Thanksgiving. She had slight discomfort with the IV during infusion, but basically all went as normal, and this being the short phase, we were at Kowloon's for lunch by eleven thirty and home by one thirty, where she immediately went for a needed four-hour nap. Mary doesn't sleep well again partly because she is so worried. Of course, she has never slept well, and this is just added pressure. One great thing this time around is her appetite, either because the chemo is having a different effect or the food in New England is just so darn good. Once this cancer is defeated, we will have to watch our midsections. Tomorrow morning will see us off to Boston again for the booster shot that helps the white blood cells.

11-09-2007   today took us back to Dana-Farber for the booster shot, which can only be given twenty-four hours after the last chemotherapy infusion. As usual, Mary was up in the middle of the night, but yesterday left her really tired and she was very early to bed, as she is today. Most of what I write is related to her treatment, but there is another side just as important, and that is her frame of mind and spirit. We all know she has spirit. However, since coming home, that spirit has grown and her support base has grown as well. This week Mary's son, Chris, called to see how she was doing and ended the call by telling her he loved her. And of course, Stephanie is just wonderful. And of course, her brother's visit from Seattle as well as the numerous cousins and family she has here. My children call regularly, and so many loving, caring friends in Florida and here provide a level of support that can't be measured medically. Mary has a real big war to win. She wins some battles and loses others. The blocked artery let her win the battle with smoking, but she is losing that war wanting them back again. So remember in our prayers to ask him to take that urge away because chemotherapy does not like cigarettes. But all in all she is doing great, her appetite is strong, taste buds haven't been damaged this time, and we have learned so much on what to look for. The next cycle begins on November 23, and after that cycle she will have a CT scan to determine the effect of the chemo.

11-23-2007   Mary and Peggy Sue at Dana-Farber at 1:15 PM to have IV fitted, then visit with the oncologist, who had encouraging words for us, "There is a 70 percent chance the chemo will shrink the tumor to allow surgery, but if God forbid it doesn't, we have other options, which we will discuss after the CT Scan on December 10." Mary has had some new pains lately and thought she could only take ibuprofen, but the oncologist told her he forbid it and Aleve, she can only take Tylenol. He said the Gemzar (one of the chemo drugs) would cause the pain. Her hemoglobin was low, which is the reason she has been so tired. He ordered a shot that she received during the chemo administration. At two forty-five, Mary and Peggy Sue were back at the clinic for the chemo administration. With the help of the nurse, I persuaded Mary to have a flu shot as well. She returns next Friday, November 30, for the second treatment of this third cycle, then Saturday for the white blood cell shot. The CT scan results on the tenth of December will be discussed with the doctor on December 14, and the next steps will be decided.

Oh, Peggy Sue is a Build-A-Bear wearing her pink bathrobe with a hood sent by Mary's brother and sister-in-law to help in the healing process. These little things, which really are *big*, help with health and spirit.

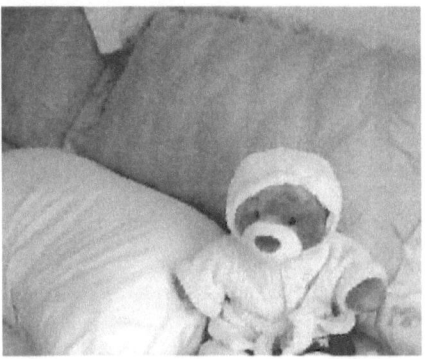

Peggy Sue

11-27-2007 Mary had a mammogram at Brigham and Women's Hospital today.

11-30-2007 Mary has been weak and had pain with her legs most of the week. We have seen this before, last year, around the time of the third cycle, which today was the second visit of the third cycle. We needed a wheelchair as we did in Florida last year, but not quite as bad as then. Last week her hemoglobin was low and she had a shot, but that wasn't the problem this time. She needed a blood transfusion, which also happened last year in Florida. Today she received two units, and tomorrow we need to go back for the white cell booster shot. So what is usually a two-hour visit on the second visit turned out to be the whole day. We discussed the junk she was told showed up in her lungs and were informed it was just that, junk from smoking and so far no indication that more cancer is there. Mary continues to be depressed, which is understandable under the circumstances. The wheelchair was not needed after the transfusion.

12-06-2007 results of mammogram came back with no evidence of new cancer.

12-14-2007 today we received an early Christmas present, a miracle, in fact. We traveled to Dana-Farber in Boston to get the results of the CT scan performed on Monday, the tenth. We were hoping to find out the tumor had shrunk so surgery could be performed. We also expected to continue with the fourth cycle of chemo for that shrinking process. The nurse practitioner informed us the cancer is completely gone, not shrunk, *gone*. A little while later, Mary's oncologist came in the room and confirmed it. There doesn't appear to be cancer anywhere in Mary's body. Mary's oncologist will meet with the urologist and discuss the next step. They may want to remove her bladder for insurance of no reoccurrence. The fourth cycle of chemo is cancelled. We drove home on cloud nine, thanking God for such a miracle because even the doctors were surprised. We will continue to pray that we have seen the last of cancer.

12-17-2007 Mary's oncologist called to say he had met with the urologist and they are weighing the next step, either radiation or surgery. The doctors want to be as certain as they can that the cancer doesn't return. Laurie Appleby told Mary last Friday she also has some emphysema. The doctors are also concerned for the effect on her aneurysm, which was at 4.6 centimeters in the last measurement. Good old cigarettes.

12-18-2007 the oncology office called to give Mary appointments for January 10, 2008. First for a vascular consultation at 9:10 AM, then for a radiation consult with the radiation doctor. Sort of looks like the next step will be radiation. The vascular consultation is for her aneurysm, I assume. Mary is still understandably very tired. She, however, is not as sick as she was the first time around, and we hope she will be her own ambitious self real soon. For now she gets to enjoy the holidays and her grandchildren.

01-10-2008, 9:10 AM—Mary had an appointment with a doctor in the Division of Vascular and Endovascular Surgery at Brigham and Women's Hospital for a consultation regarding her aortic aneurysm. The doctor explained that he had looked at the CT scan for the lymph node tumor and determined the aneurysm is about 4.4 centimeters instead of 4.6 centimeters. Mary asked the doctor why they would not consider surgery until the size reached 5 centimeters. He explained the mortality rate for this type of surgery is not very good but the risk at 5 centimeters was just about the same, so that was how the size for surgery is determined, that is, when the risk factor is about the same. He did explain though, there are new procedures that are not as risky. He liked my report and said I can find the details of what he told us on the Internet, which I will do, and I will include them in www.maryshealth.htm. He will order a CT scan for just the aneurysm and meet with the other doctors to determine if the radiation treatment will affect the size and whether or not they should operate. He told Mary her situation is not the normal, off-the-street type of situation and would be treated specially. There are two major techniques for the repair of aortic aneurysms. The traditional open surgical operation is an option available to most patients. This is a major surgical procedure performed through an abdominal incision. The aneurysm is repaired by replacing the diseased segment of the aorta with a strong and durable artificial graft, which is sewn in its place. Although this is a major operation, it is an extremely durable and effective way to treat abdominal aortic aneurysms. More recently, newer catheter-based technologies allow minimally invasive treatment of aortic aneurysms. In this technique, small incisions are made in the groin, and using x-ray control, catheters are placed internally up into the aorta. The catheters are then used to deploy aortic stent grafts, which anchor above and below the aneurysm, thus repairing the aneurysm from the inside. This procedure is generally well tolerated and results in a shorter hospital stay, generally about two days. Following placement of an aortic stent graft, patients require ongoing long-term follow-up with CT scans to ensure that the grafts are functioning properly. There are certain anatomic requirements for safe placement of an aortic stent graft, and not all patients have appropriate anatomy for this procedure. *Mortality rate* is the number of deaths in a place or group compared with the total number of people in that place or group The inpatient mortality rate for AAA repair at Brigham and Women's Hospital is 0 percent, which is better than both the national average (1.73 percent) and expected (4.85 percent) rates. All rates refer to the twelve-month period ending on June 30, 2007. At 2:00 PM, Mary had an appointment with an MD (clinician and researcher) for genitourinary cancer, medical oncology, radiation oncology at Dana-Farber Cancer Institute. First, the doctor assured Mary the radiation treatment will not have any effect on the aneurysm. She is trying to schedule an appointment for Monday afternoon, January 14, for a CT scan of the area where the latest tumors were located. During the scan, as part of the procedure, she will draw up Mary's treatment dosage. She will be receiving radiation treatments five days a week for six weeks and chemotherapy with cisplatin every Monday. The doctor added that Mary's oncologist and urologist do not feel surgery is necessary at this time. This doctor also used a term no one has used before: the cancer is in remission. She said their goal is to make sure it stays in remission.

Radiation Oncology

01-15-2008 at 2:00 PM today, Mary had a series of CT scans to be used
in mapping out the radiation program for her. They put at
least two tattoos on her lower body for the target area of the
radiation. We are still having trouble getting her original CT
scan from the doctors in Boca but are getting closer. We must
have those scans within the next four weeks. On January 31,
2008, the radiation treatment will begin, but actually that day
will more than likely be a trial run and the actual radiation will
begin on Monday, February 4. The treatment will consist of
about twenty minutes of radiation, five days a week for about
six weeks. Each week will begin with chemotherapy (cisplatin
administered). They encourage people to keep a normal schedule
and to maintain their usual level of activity during treatment as
long as it is comfortable. Fatigue is a common side effect of
radiation therapy and may occur at any time. Incorporating a
rest period or nap into the day is often helpful. It is important to
keep oneself hydrated throughout the treatment. At least eight
ounces of water, juice, Gatorade, etc., should be taken each
day. A regular multivitamin is fine to take during treatment,
but high doses of vitamin or supplements should be avoided.
In general, antioxidants (selenium, vitamins C and E) are not
recommended during radiation therapy, as they interfere with
the changes necessary for the radiation to work. During radiation
therapy, the skin in the treatment area may become reddened,
dry, irritated, or itchy. These reactions are temporary and usually
subside within a few weeks of completion of treatment. Use
warm water and gentle soap on the area being treated (Dove,

Basis, Pears, Pure & Natural, Neutrogena, and Oil of Olay, for example). Deodorant soaps and antiperspirants should not be used. Perfumes, cosmetics, or powders should be avoided in the treatment area. Do not expose the treated area to extreme temperatures, like ice packs, heating pads, hot tubs, or saunas, and sun exposure should be limited.

XII—Radiation Treatment to Begin

01-31-2008   a radiation trial run was conducted today, providing Mary with what to expect. A total of twenty-five treatments will begin Monday, February 4, 2008. She will be at the hospital in Boston five days a week. Only two days will be skipped, Friday, February 8, and Monday, February 18. We do not as yet have a schedule for the chemo treatment.

02-05-2008   today was the second day of radiation treatments (ten minutes every day). Mary met with the radiation doctor after the session (she will have this meeting every Tuesday). The doctor informed us she thinks she still sees some cancer and that is the reason for the radiation. After the radiation tomorrow, Mary will have some more chemo, about four hours of treatment. She can expect this chemo probably once a week. On Thursday she will see her primary care doctor. All the doctors at Brigham and Women's Hospital and Dana-Farber work together as a team on all of Mary's medical problems. They also offer social services help, but thank God Mary is still coping pretty well. Toughie!

02-06-2008   after the ten-minute radiation treatment, Mary had four hours of chemo, the old cisplatin drug again. She will get the chemo every two weeks while she is getting her radiation treatments. At the end she will have another series of CT scans to check status. Tomorrow before the radiation treatment, she will see her primary care doctor.

02-07-2008   a 10:00 AM appointment with primary care doctor went well with nothing new to discuss and a renewal of Lipitor prescription. The secretary from the office of the vascular and endovascular surgeon called to request information regarding the side of the carotid artery to allow an ultrasound in the near future. Nausea set in yesterday after the chemo and again today, even though the treatment today was the radiation at ten thirty. Tomorrow is a day off, no doctors, no treatment, just staying at home and watching the snow fall.

02-12-2008 after the daily radiation treatment, Mary met with the doctor in radiation oncology, which she does every Tuesday. The doctor told her everything looks real good. Hopefully meaning the treatment is working. Mary still gets very tired, but input like this helps pep her up.

02-16-2008 yesterday, February 15, was the eighth radiation treatment. There has been one chemo treatment. Monday is a holiday, so the day is off, but Tuesday is a full day with radiation and chemotherapy. We were told the treatment would make Mary tired, and it has. Fortunately though, the appetite problem has not reoccurred, nor the sores in the mouth. She, however, has no energy, so most activity will be put on hold until after the treatments are finished, about March 12.

02-19-2008 this is being written at Dana-Farber while Mary is receiving her chemotherapy (cisplatin). She had radiation at ten thirty and now at 3:00 PM is just finishing her chemo. Met with radiation doctor this morning after radiation, and she is not seeing anything there now. Met with her oncologist before the chemo treatment, and he said everything is looking good and this just might be the last chemo. He also told Mary there is nothing showing on the CT scans. He further told her the hearing loss is caused by the chemo drugs and is common. We need to extend our insurance, but because of preexisting conditions, that may be difficult after December unless she is considered disabled. The doctor says she is and he will sign necessary papers to confirm that. Prayers are being answered all over the place.

02-26-2008   although the radiation and chemotherapy are wearing Mary down, leaving her very tired, she did get some more encouraging news from the radiation oncology doctor today. She was told her blood counts are better than those of most people without cancer. Tomorrow will be a long day for her with radiation at ten thirty followed at one thirty with another CT scan.

03-04-2008   another long day at Dana-Farber, but well worth the time. We were scheduled to be at Dana-Farber at 8:00 AM to prepare for infusion and to meet with the nurse practitioner in the oncology department at eight thirty. Traffic was bad, so we were about forty minutes late. Mary's white cell and platelet counts were down, so Laurie scheduled a blood transfusion after the regular ten-thirty radiation and Tuesday meeting with the radiation oncology doctor, who told Mary everything is looking good and she will have six more radiation treatments. Chemo infusion was cancelled and replaced with blood transfusion of two units, which returned blood pressure to near normal. The cell and platelet counts were the major cause of her being so tired.

03-05-2008   Mary called and cancelled her appointment due to real bad weather. We will be back on schedule tomorrow and still have six more treatments. After that she probably won't need to see a doctor until April.

03-17-2008   it is St. Patrick's Day 2008, and Mary has officially been sick 518 days. She is tired, but any lesser individual would be finished. She is now entering another cycle of loss of appetite, but we are pushing food at her and she has nausea pills, which will, hopefully, help us. With any luck there should only be about ten days of radiation left. Then she can start the road back to normal. And with God's help, the cancer will be gone.

03-25-2008   Mary met with the radiation oncology doctor after her radiation treatment today and was told she is doing very well. Her radiation treatment is scheduled to end in two days (Thursday, the twenty-seventh). If all goes well, she doesn't have to see any doctors or medical personnel until her appointment with her oncologist on May 20.

05-20-2008 Mary's oncologist said the CT scan was clean and the next appointment will be in four months to include an MRI and another CT scan. He also said to make an appointment with the urologist for a look inside the bladder, to contact the primary for another blood checkup when we return from Italy. There is already a scheduled cardiologist appointment on July 21 to check the carotid artery and aneurysm. Today due to low blood counts (normal is 34 to 45, and today it was at 20), a three-hour blood transfusion was performed, providing two units of blood.

07-01-2008 Jesus said to the two blind men, "Believe ye that I am able to do this?" Then he touched their eyes, saying, "According to your faith be it unto you," and their eyes were opened (Matthew 9:28–29). Maybe not quite this dramatic, but just as important to us. Through the faith of so many who have prayed, Mary received more good news today. The urologist told her after the cystoscopy was finished that the treatment appears to have worked. *There is no sign of tumor.* Thanks so much to all who have prayed for this moment, but of course we will all continue to pray because this disease is a nasty one that likes to make repeat appearances. Mary told the doctor she went high up visiting the Vatican with her prayers. He said it seems to have worked.

07-21-2008 Mary had an ultrasound of her abdomen at twelve forty-five, Monday, July 21, 2008. Then at 2:00 PM in the vascular lab, she had an ultrasound of the carotid arteries. Then at 3:10 PM she saw the vascular and endovascular surgeon. The arteries are clean, so no problems there, thanks to giving up the cigarettes. The abdominal aortic aneurysm has grown some, which is normal but is now at a point where she will need to be checked again in about three months. Not all aneurysms need an operation; some aneurysms may be suitable for treatment by a new method in which the graft is threaded up into the aortic aneurysm through a small incision in each groin. At this point, Mary is eligible for this procedure. The next appointments are for a MRI and CT scan on September 10, with a follow-up visit on the sixteenth with the oncologist. For now then, it seems the cancer is gone, the arteries are clean, and the aneurysm is under control. Mary, of course, is concerned and very worried about the aneurysm. She does not and will not talk about it.

07-25-2008 with the cancer on the back burner for now and the carotid arteries clear, it may be a good time to revisit the other danger: the abdominal aortic aneurysm. Below are a few definitions that might explain why Mary is scared again. Abdominal aortic aneurysm (AAA) is a vascular disease with life-threatening implications. If you have a family history of abdominal aortic aneurysm or have smoked at least one hundred cigarettes in your lifetime, you are considered at risk. Surgery is recommended for patients with aneurysms bigger than 5.5 centimeters in diameter and aneurysms that rapidly increase in size. The goal is to perform surgery before complications or symptoms develop. There are two approaches to surgery. In a traditional (open) repair, a large cut is made in your abdomen. The abnormal vessel is replaced with a graft made of synthetic material, such as Dacron. The other approach is called endovascular stent grafting. An endovascular stent graft is a tube made of metal mesh that helps support the artery. Small hollow tubes called catheters are inserted through arteries in your groin. The stent graft is sent through a catheter and permanently placed into the artery. Endovascular stent grafting can be done without making a large cut in your abdomen, so you may get well faster. However, not all patients with abdominal aortic aneurysms can have this type of surgery. Outlook (prognosis)—the outcome is usually good if an experienced surgeon repairs the aneurysm before it ruptures. However, less than 40 percent of patients survive a ruptured abdominal aneurysm. Prevention exercise, eating well, and avoiding tobacco reduce the risk of developing aneurysms. Get regular physical exams. If you have any risk factors, insist upon a screening abdominal aortic ultrasound.

XIII—The Cancer Is Gone Again

09-16-2008   a visit to the oncologist to confirm the MRI and CT scan on the tenth still showed no cancer. The next CT scan and MRI will be done on January 21, 2009.

11-10-2008   saw the vascular and endovascular surgeon about the abdominal aortic aneurysm. He expects to perform an endovascular stent graft in June 2009.

11-25-2008   a 10:00 AM appointment with Mary's primary care doctor went well.

01-23-2009   Dana-Farber, blood work at ten fifteen, MRI at eleven fifteen, and CT scan at 1:20 PM.

01-27-2009   oncologist office called to say the MRI and CT scan show no sign of the cancer. Good news, but the abdominal aortic aneurysm has grown to 5.1 centimeters, so the vascular and endovascular surgeon needs to be told. Since we will have insurance again on February 1, he will probably schedule the endovascular stent grafting procedure.

03-31-2009   Mary's urologist told her after the cystoscopy was finished that the treatment appears to still be working. The bladder is still clear. Next up is blood work with the primary care doctor on May 26, 2009, in preparation for the endovascular stent grafting procedure in June. Scheduled to see the vascular and endovascular surgeon on June 8 (postponed until October).

06-3-2009   met with Mary's oncologist at Dana-Farber, finding out the MRI and CT scan show no sign of the cancer. Next cancer check will be in October.

09-01-2009   Mary's urologist told her after the cystoscopy was finished that the treatment appears to still be working. The bladder is still clear. Next cystoscopy will be in six months.

09-29-2009   the vascular and endovascular surgeon said the last review he did showed the aneurysm had not grown and was still at 4.8 centimeters. An additional CT scan to this doctor's specifications will be performed on September 30 when the regular MRI and CT scan to check on cancer is performed. Will see Mary's oncologist on October 6 for cancer results, and the vascular and endovascular surgeon will call after the CT scan to inform of any decisions on his performing any procedures. He told us he has performed hundreds of these procedures.

10-6-2009   met with Mary's oncologist at Dana-Farber, finding out the MRI and CT scan show no sign of the cancer. Next cancer check will be in February 2010. Her oncologist also read the vascular and endovascular surgeon's notes on the aneurysm and said there was no change, it has not grown.

10-13-2009   the vascular and endovascular surgeon called to inform us that the aneurysm has not grown, which is, of course, good news. However, he had a little bad news. It seems Mary's veins are too small to perform the stent procedure when the time comes, that time being, of course, when and if it grows. As of this date, we will be rechecking during the February cancer checks. If the vascular and endovascular surgeon determines at that time surgery is warranted, a traditional (open) repair, a large cut will be made in the abdomen. The abnormal vessel will be replaced with a graft made of synthetic material, such as Dacron. The outcome is usually good if an experienced surgeon repairs the aneurysm before it ruptures. In the meantime, exercise, eat well, and avoid tobacco to reduce the risk of the aneurysm growing.

02-01-2010 CT, 11:30 AM chest standard, Dana-Farber radiology, MRI at
12:15 PM for abdomen and pelvis.

02-03-2010 Mary had blood work at Elliot in Londonderry for Dana-Farber
because her potassium level was up in the blood work performed
on the first. About one and a half hours later, Dana-Farber called
to say the potassium level was back to normal.

02-09-2010 remember Tony the Tiger from the Esso days? Today our Tony
the Tiger, Mary's oncologist, said "G-R-E-A-T" when asked the
results of last week's CT scan and MRI. The appointments are
now moved to every six months. The final step in a clean bill of
health right now is the *cystoscopy* for a picture inside the bladder.
That will be scheduled in March.

XIX—Pelvic Fracture

02-17-2010 Mary had severe pain in her abdomen last year caused by fractures in the pelvic area resulting from the radiation. She was given pain medication to ease the pain until the fractures self-healed. About six weeks ago, the pain returned and her oncologist recommended an orthopedic surgeon who saw her today. He explained the radiation was done just behind the hip joint where the fracture is shown on the MRI. He further said she will just have to let it heal itself with time. Also, if she requires pain medication, she will need to contact her primary care doctor. On March 31 another CT scan will be done to determine status.

The orthopedic surgeon explained using a skeleton of the pelvis. He said the bladder is directly behind the spot I have marked with red. The radiation would have been applied directly to the bladder, and on the MRI picture he showed us the fracture was just about where I have the red. That is why he thinks the fracture was caused by the radiation and why surgery will not be required. Only time can heal the fracture.

03-23-2010 Mary's urologist told her after the cystoscopy was finished that the treatment appears to still be working. The bladder is still clear. Next cystoscopy will be in six months.

03-31-2010 CT Scan at Brigham and Women's Hospital at 10:15 AM, followed at 11:00 AM with an appointment the orthopedic surgeon, who explained from the CT scan that it appears healing is taking place but is real slow and for us to expect probably six more months to heal. It is important to schedule a bone density test through her primary care doctor.

04-15-2010   bone density done at Brigham and Women's in Chestnut Hill. Mary's primary care doctor will be seen on April 23 to discuss the results.

08-05-2010   CT scan only this trip, MRI not needed.

08-12-2010   met with the nurse practitioner in the oncology department who reported no return of cancer. She also said the pain in the hip was not from the cracked pelvis, but from osteoporosis. She set up an appointment with a different orthopedic doctor for September 8, 2010 (the previous surgeon has moved on to other things). Also no change in the growth of the aneurysm.

09-08-2010   met with a new orthopedic surgeon at Brigham and Women's Hospital. While reviewing x-rays, a small break in the hip was seen. This doctor reasons this is the cause of the severe pain. This doctor has suggested full hip replacement using procedure 1 below. He also suggested we get a second opinion. He recommended several doctors.

Hip replacement surgery

Total joint replacement involves surgery to replace the ends of both bones in a damaged joint to create new joint surfaces.

Total hip replacement surgery replaces the upper end of the thighbone (femur) with a metal ball and resurfaces the hip socket in the pelvic bone with a metal shell and plastic liner.

Total hip replacement surgery replaces damaged cartilage with new joint material in a step-by-step process.

Doctors may attach replacement joints to the bones with or without cement.

- 1—Cemented joints are attached to the existing bone with cement, which acts as a glue and attaches the artificial joint to the bone.

- 2—Uncemented joints are attached using a porous coating that is designed to allow the bone to adhere to the artificial joint. Over time, new bone grows and fills up the openings in the porous coating, attaching the joint to the bone.

12-15-2010 met with the chief of orthopedic surgery at Brigham and Women's Hospital for a second opinion. The chief agrees with the orthopedic surgeon that a full hip is needed. A presurgery appointment is made for December 22, 2010, with the orthopedic surgeon.

12-22-2010 met with the orthopedic surgeon at Brigham and Women's

Hospital to schedule surgery. However, an infection appeared from the blood work done on the fifteenth. Tomorrow, December 23, at noon, nuclear medicine bone scan 3 phase is scheduled. There will be an injection at noon, followed three hours later with the bone scan. We also have to call the vascular and endovascular surgeon to see how the aneurysm might be affected. An appointment is scheduled with the orthopedic surgeon on the twenty-ninth at ten fifteen to discuss all test results. If everything is a go, that go will be surgery sometime during the first week in January.

Mary has been in severe pain since sometime in October. The primary care doctor provided prescriptions for one of the weaker drugs that did not help. Complaining to anyone that would listen about the pain and lack of medical concern brought progress today. The orthopedic surgeon wrote a stronger prescription. Hopefully, it will help because she cannot eat or sleep because of the pain.

12-23-2010 we were accepted early at 11:30 AM. The injection took only a few minutes, and we were told to return at 2:00 PM for the bone scan. The bone scan ended at about 3:30 PM. Of course, no results will be known until the twenty-ninth when we see the orthopedic surgeon again. A message was sent to the vascular and endovascular surgeon, but we have no idea whether he will call us or the orthopedic surgeon.

12-24-2010 not having heard from the vascular and endovascular surgeon (this is the aneurysm doctor), Mary called his office only to find out he is on vacation until January. This, of course, could create further delays.

12-29-2010 arrived at ten fifteen and was met in the hall by the orthopedic surgeon who said he now wanted a back x-ray, so off we went to radiation. After the x-ray the orthopedic surgeon explained that since the hip pain has subsided and the pain has now moved to the back, more tests will need to be performed to make absolutely sure the hip replacement is required. So at 8:00 AM on January 12, 2011, an MRI will be done of the back, then on to Dr. Ferrone at nine fifteen. Now this seems a lot of this and that, but as the doctor pointed out, we would hate to do a complete hip replacement and find out that was not the cause of the pain. All the treatments for cancer are wonderful, but they do have unexpected side effects.

Vascular and Endovascular Surgery

UPDATE: January 13, 2011

01-06-2011   Mary received a call that another back x-ray was required and
scheduled at 1:00 PM on January 6, 2011. It turned out to be
the dreaded biopsy, and she became very faint when they told
her. However, because she has lost so much weight, it was much
easier than expected.

01-13-2011   Mary went in to the examining room with the vascular and
endovascular surgeon (this is the aneurysm doctor), alone this
time, so my report is hearsay. It seems the aneurysm has grown.
She also informed me the other doctors will not do anything
until the aneurysm is fixed. The MRI and blood work scheduled
for yesterday were done at 3:00 PM today. The vascular and
endovascular surgeon will review the results and determine his
course of action to fix the aneurysm. Although I wasn't there, it
sounds to me like the fix is near at hand. The appointment with
the orthopedic surgeon is schedule for 3:00 K on the nineteenth.
(Again note, nothing will be done until the aneurysm is fixed.)

In human anatomy, the **vertebral column**) is a column usually
consisting of 24 articulating **vertebrae**,[1], and 9 fused vertebrae
in the sacrum and the coccyx. It is situated in the dorsal aspect
of the torso, separated by intervertebral discs. It houses and
protects the spinal cord in its spinal canal.

01-19-2011   the orthopedic surgeon said they found a crack in the lumbar

L1, and this could be causing the pain in connection with the aneurysm.

After the aneurysm is fixed, if the pain is still there, it can usually be corrected with back braces in time. If not, they fill with a sort of cement. He said the biopsy was not a biopsy, but they injected a pain reliever to see if the pain would slacken; since it didn't, they are now fairly certain a full hip replacement is not needed.

The orthopedic surgeon said he will call the vascular and endovascular surgeon to discuss the situation and perhaps get the aneurysm procedure started.

Mary asked to switch medicine back to Vicodin because the oxycodone was making her sick. I explained that originally he has said if half a pill didn't work, she should use a whole pill, and it didn't work. This created legal and insurance problems, so could he make it one every four hours And he did, 180 pills for thirty days.

01-25-2011   Mary had a very successful visit with her primary care doctor, who promised to do all she could to get things moving.

This afternoon the vascular and endovascular surgeon called me to explain what is happening. The full operation is a painful experience with a very long recovery/rehab process. They have been using an alternative procedure (which seems to be a sort of detour). The operation requires careful planning with special charts. He has already started the planning, and the charts are done. In the plan if there is a problem, he can stop and go to a full operation, but in more than ten years, he has not had to do this. Mary probably has a 20 percent chance of being a patient this might be necessary because of her clogged arteries below the aneurysm, but in any case she will still be fixed, just have the longer recovery. The next step is for the vascular and endovascular surgeon to talk to oncology at Dana-Farber and make sure the cancer is gone. He said if she still had cancer, there wouldn't be much point in making her suffer through this operation. He said he will be in touch soon.

Although it might seem dire, I am happy that they check every possibility, no matter how remote.

Updates are sketchy from the above date in January until the April date below. However, there are some facts from insurance explanation of benefits.

02-08-2011 the abdominal aortic aneurysm operation was performed successfully by the vascular and endovascular surgeon today.

02-14-2011 Mary started receiving skilled nursing and physical therapy from home health care professionals.

02-24-2011 after the follow-up appointment the vascular and endovascular surgeon with, Mary's husband, John, suffered congestive heart failure and was rushed to Massachusetts General Hospital, where a team of cardiologists saved his life. However, he would be out for the next eight weeks.

03-01-2011 Mary taken to the emergency room at Southern New Hampshire Medical Center in Nashua, New Hampshire, with an infection.

03-08-2011 Mary was readmitted to Brigham and Women's Hospital in Boston.

03-10-2011 Mary is again at the emergency room of Brigham and Women's Hospital.

04-18-2011 Mary is again at the emergency room of Brigham and Women's Hospital.

04-24-2011 Mary has been back in the hospital for a week now and, hopefully, will come home today, Easter Sunday. She developed a fistula (attachment of the gallbladder to the lower intestine). This is often caused by abdominal surgery. She also developed an ulcer from the Advil and Aleve she was taking for the pain in her spine.

Mary had been warned by her oncologist not to take Advil and Aleve. However, due to the circumstance of her illness and her husband's absence due to his illness, she was given that medicine because of the difficulty in picking up prescriptions in person from her primary care doctor.

Once the fistula is cleared up and the ulcer is gone (probably four to six weeks), her gallbladder will be removed so this can't happen again (http://en.wikipedia.org/wiki/Fistula).

05-07-2011 we don't have a lot of news regarding Mary's health but may have quite a bit after she sees the surgeon who will remove her gallbladder. On Tuesday, May, the tenth, Mary has a scheduled CT scan early in the morning. She will then meet with the surgeon at noon, hopefully, to schedule the surgery to remove it. In the meantime, the liquid diet is driving her nuts and causing more weight loss. She is now under one hundred pounds. She is naturally very depressed, and that is no surprise. Any lesser person would have been depressed years ago. I don't know if it is the Irish blood or the Portuguese, but she is certainly a fighter. Mary has been through a lot for nearly six years now.

Surgical Oncology

05-10-2011   Mary had her CT scan today, and the fistula hasn't healed yet. She has another CT scan and visit with the oncology surgeon in about four weeks. The gallbladder cannot be removed until the fistula is healed. The doctor did, however, allow her to start eating again. When we finished, we headed straight for the Venezia Restaurant and veal parmesan.

06-14-2011   Mary had her appointment with the oncology surgeon today, and the fistula hasn't healed yet. The doctor said they will have to remove it with the gallbladder and explained in some detail with pictures he drew just what would be involved. He said there are two types of surgery but Mary's situation being unique would require the second type, open gallbladder surgery, which I found on Web MD and captured most of what he told us, and I have that explanation below. I have highlighted the portion that appears to apply to Mary.

Laparoscopic gallbladder surgery is the most common surgery done to remove the gallbladder. In this type of surgery, a doctor inserts a lighted viewing instrument called a laparoscope and surgical tools into your abdomen through several small cuts (incisions). This type of surgery is very safe, and people who have it usually recover enough in about one week to go back to work or to their normal routines.

Open gallbladder surgery involves one larger incision through which the gallbladder is removed. It may be done if laparoscopic surgery is not an option or when complications are found during laparoscopic surgery. Most open surgeries occur after trying to do a laparoscopic cholecystectomy. Open surgery also may be the best choice if the blood won't clot well, the anatomy is not normal, or there is too much scarring from previous surgery.

Recovery is much faster and less painful after laparoscopic surgery than after open surgery.

- The hospital stay after laparoscopic surgery is shorter than after open surgery. In general people go home the same day or the next day compared with 2 to 4 days for open surgery.

- Recovery is faster after laparoscopic surgery.

- You will spend less time away from work and other activities after laparoscopic surgery (about a week to 10 days compared with 4 to 6 weeks for open surgery).

06-20-2011 pre-op at 1:00 PM, Tuesday, June 21, 2011.

These results are best explained in Mary's own words.

The nurse in pre-op told Mary she has never seen anything like my gallbladder scenario, and she has been doing it for nine years. Mary commented, "Yeah, that's me. I always have to have something unusual. So that makes me a wee bit nervous. My doctor didn't say a word about it except he had done one like mine . . . just one. Why can't I have a normal enlarged gallbladder? So I guess I am out of commission for the summer since they have to open me up."

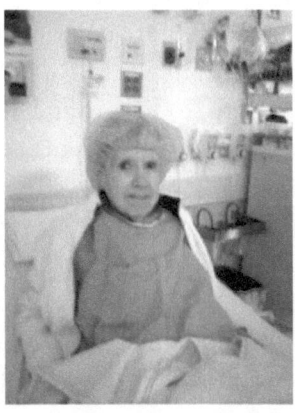

06-23-2011 Surgery, 7:30 AM

The oncology surgeon called and said she did great. There weren't any complications and she wasn't as bad as thought earlier. No sign of cancer that he can see. Gallbladder is removed and sent for lab work, which will take a week or more. Surgery scheduled to be five hours but obviously much less.

06-24-2011 at 3:00 PM I just returned from visiting Mary at BWH. She seems to be doing well, a lot of pain, but that is to be expected. They have given her a button that allows her to regulate her pain medicine. When I spoke with her at 9:00 AM, she said the pain was a 10 on a level from 1 to 10, but when I got to the hospital at ten thirty, she said it was down to an eight. She has good nurses, and they got her up into a chair to sit for a while. She is expecting physical therapy this afternoon. She kicked me out at one because she said her worry about my driving home was worse than me not being there. The doctor had not been in yet.

06-29-2011 she is much better today, already on solid foods. Brigham's physical therapist worked with her a little while I was there today. She has been accepted by a rehab center and may be moved there by ambulance tomorrow (Thursday). After I left her, I went to the rehab center to see the people who cared for me and let them know I had recommended them because of the great care I received. They are looking forward to helping her.

06-30-2011 Mary arrived at rehab today at three fifteen to begin her rehab. She looked a little better, said she had no pain but was very tired. She is on a regular diet and had a cheese steak sandwich delivered for supper but was too worn out to eat. The physician's assistant came by to see her around 6:00 PM. I saw many people I met in my stay, mainly the physical therapists who assured me they will get her up and walking. The rehab center is only a few minutes away, so we can spend time with her, if it helps in the recovery.

07-12-2011 on Mary's visit with the surgeon on Tuesday, he was concerned with her pain and lack of healing. She is again admitted to

Brigham and Women's Hospital. Due to lack of nourishment, fluid had built up around the fistula. A tube was placed to drain off the fluid. Mary's oncologist came over from Dana-Farber to see Mary, but she was having the tube inserted at the time. He informed me that the oncology surgeon found a growth of some sort in her back, which will be checked to make sure the cancer has not returned.

07-19-2011   Mary was told today there is no problem with the growth on her back. She is walking just a little but really suffering (understandably) depression over such a long illness. She, however, is still a trooper and working to get better.

07-20-2011   a resident doctor explained the three drain tubes for fluid (third one added this morning). The fluid from the fistula is leaking into her other organs, liver, etc. This is the fluid mentioned before and created by lack of nourishment, and the two tubes inserted before were not draining it all. During the process this morning, a lot of fluid was suctioned off (close to a half liter), and hopefully, the new tube will drain the rest. The wound cannot heal until the fluid is gone.

07-24-2011, 12:13 PM, Sunday, July 24, 2011—not too much change this morning. Mary is real tired today and, as usual, objecting to everything. Annette called from Rhode Island (a friend from Florida) and is going to come see her; she objects, but Annette is still coming. An aide fixed her hair so she will look good, but since she was told she was getting visitors, she has a scowl on her face. She said the oncology surgeon was in before I arrived but had nothing new to tell her. I do believe there is more progress because she is moving much better without help (and complaining more).

It was a month yesterday since this last operation. Twelve days since she was admitted this time. Yesterday we were told she is about ready for rehab again.

08-03-2011   Mary is still in the hospital but improving slowly. She is now walking around the nurse pod three times a day. She only has one tube and the IV line for her nourishment. fluid is still leaking into her body but has slowed somewhat. She will not heal until all the fluid is gone.

08-08-2011 today Mary was moved to Spaulding Rehab in Cambridge. Spaulding is also part of the Partners network, which includes Brigham and Women's Hospital and Massachusetts General Hospital.

08-11-2011 an x-ray at Spaulding showed the hip fracture never healed as she was told by the orthopedic surgeon. Therefore, I now refer to him as Phony. Someone remarked there are others within the facility who feel somewhat the same, but no names were given. I also believe the arrogance of that doctor and his ignoring of the pain Mary had to endure contributed to the development of the fistula.

08-18-2011 Mary was transported to Massachusetts General Hospital to have her hip x-rayed again and to meet with a Mass General orthopedic surgeon. She had requested that further treatment should be at MGH. She saw a resident who explained to her satisfaction what to expect. Together they decided on replacement hip surgery the week after next. The surgeon whom she is still to meet that will perform the operation as part of a team. The resident who checked her will probably be part of the team as well.

Orthopedic Trauma Service

The orthopedic trauma surgeon is a leading specialist who treats orthopedic injuries of the hip and the pelvis. As chief of the Partners Orthopedic Trauma Service, he has created a care delivery system, ensuring patients receive optimal care during their recovery.

09-01-2011   Mary was transported to Massachusetts General Hospital in preparation for her full hip replacement scheduled for September 2, 2011.

09-02-2011   Mary was taken into surgery at 10:30 AM, and the resident called me in the waiting room at 3:44 PM to tell me everything went very well and she is in recovery with a brand-new hip. As I have noted in other areas, procedures at Massachusetts General Hospital appear to be much better organized, providing more efficient and professional care.

09-15-2011   Mary had x-ray of her lungs on September 13, 2011, and today the doctor at Spaulding said she had a small collapse of one lung but it was not large enough to be a worry. This was assumed to be the result of recent surgery, probably the fistula.

10-29-2011   Mary is still in Spaulding Cambridge Rehab. She is scheduled for an upper GI on Monday, the thirty-first, and a CT scan on Tuesday, November 1, to determine if she can have surgery on Thursday, November 3, to finally close the hole left by the fistula operation and stop the drain to an exterior bag. Her hip has healed, and physically she is very fit and ready to come home.

11-03-2011   at nine thirty this morning, Mary went into pre-op at Brigham and Women's Hospital for surgery by the oncology surgeon to repair the nonhealing from the fistula operation. The surgery took between four and six hours. She appeared to get through the surgery well, according to the oncology surgeon. It is expected she will be a patient at BWH for about two weeks, but then she should be discharged to go home instead of back to rehab.

11-10-2011   Mary has developed a urinary infection from the catheter (she got one here before in February). Since she is allergic to penicillin, they will be using an antibiotic from a different family and closely monitoring the effect.

11-14-2011   Mary's body is being tested with two feeds, one through a tube in her abdomen and the other the TPM through the IV line. She will have a CT scan today around 2:00 PM, and hopefully, the result she will begin very small bits of whole food. This will be the first real food to enter her body since June 22, 2011, the day before the fistula surgery (four and a half months).

11-24-2011   Thanksgiving 2011. Not where Mary wanted to be. The oncology surgeon was in and said the healing is happening. An associate of the oncology surgeon came in and checked Mary's surgery, finding one of the abdomen tubes for draining was out. He said this might not be needed anymore and told her instead of weeks she may be on oral food in days and possibly headed for the next step, which we hope is home, instead of rehab. The other tube she has is for the feeding, and of course, once she can take food orally, it too will be gone. The secret to the rest of her healing is moving about, and after all the failures, Mary is reluctant to believe that will help. The emotional drain is large after such a long return to health.

12-08-2011   Mary finally came home from Brigham and Women's Hospital on December, the third, after a very long ordeal. She is still far from well and will be tube-fed through her stomach for some time. In fact, only minutes ago, a three-month supply arrived, kind of gives everyone the idea of the seriousness of her problem.

She is getting little portions of real food, like a teaspoon or so once in a while. However, she is healing although slow. Today the home health care nurse said she is now well enough to cut back on their visits. The months ahead will be filled with many doctor visits for sure, but she is on the mend.

12-9-2011   due to dehydration from diarrhea and nausea Mary was re-admitted to Brigham and Women's Hospital.

12-16-2011 Mary was moved to rehab in Nashua, New Hampshire, yesterday afternoon. Her nausea and diarrhea problems are gone and she is eating rather normal now. This rehab is mostly for her to gain her strength again. The rehab center is only about four miles from home, and they have a pretty good physical and occupational therapy group. In addition there is an on-site beautician whom we used before to do Mary's hair. Although there is no more tube feeding, Mary still has the J-tube in her stomach for some fiber input.

12-26-2011 the day after Christmas, and I think I can safely say Mary has now started the long road to recovery. She is stronger, eating better with less nausea and making most of her decisions herself with confidence. In therapy she is climbing stairs and currently working on regaining her balance to walk without a walker.

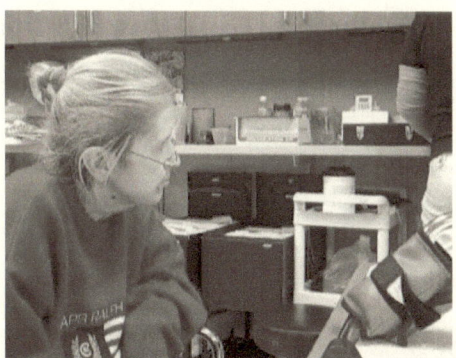

Mary looks at the portable pedaling machine used
in her occupational therapy at the rehab center.

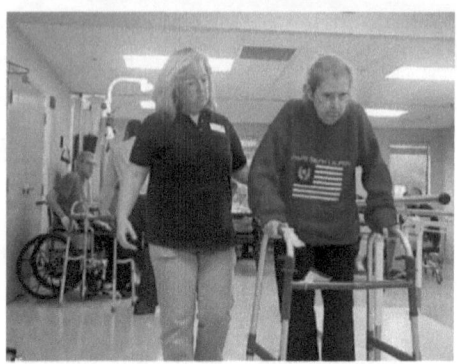

Mary walks during physical therapy and will follow with
practice for balance without the walker. After five major
surgeries in 2011, this is a major step toward recovery.

01-11-2012   Mary had a follow-up appointment with the oncology surgeon
at 1:30 PM but had to wait for one whole hour. We arrived one
hour early, so the poor kid had a two-hour wait. While waiting
she ate a considerable amount of mac and cheese. The doctor was
pleased with her progress. We arrived back at rehab in Nashua
about 4:30 PM. The nurse at rehab had talked to the doctor and
said we should set up a family meeting to begin the discharge
process for Mary. That meeting is set up for one thirty next
Wednesday, January 18. I left her around 8:00 PM to go home,
and she was quite pleased with the results of such a long day and
now looking forward to going home.

01-22-2012   Mary discharged from rehab and will finish her rehab at home.

Index